# DIABETES AND KIDNEY HEALTH COOKBOOK

## Nutrient-Packed Recipes for Managing Chronic Conditions

**Dr Lily Morgan**

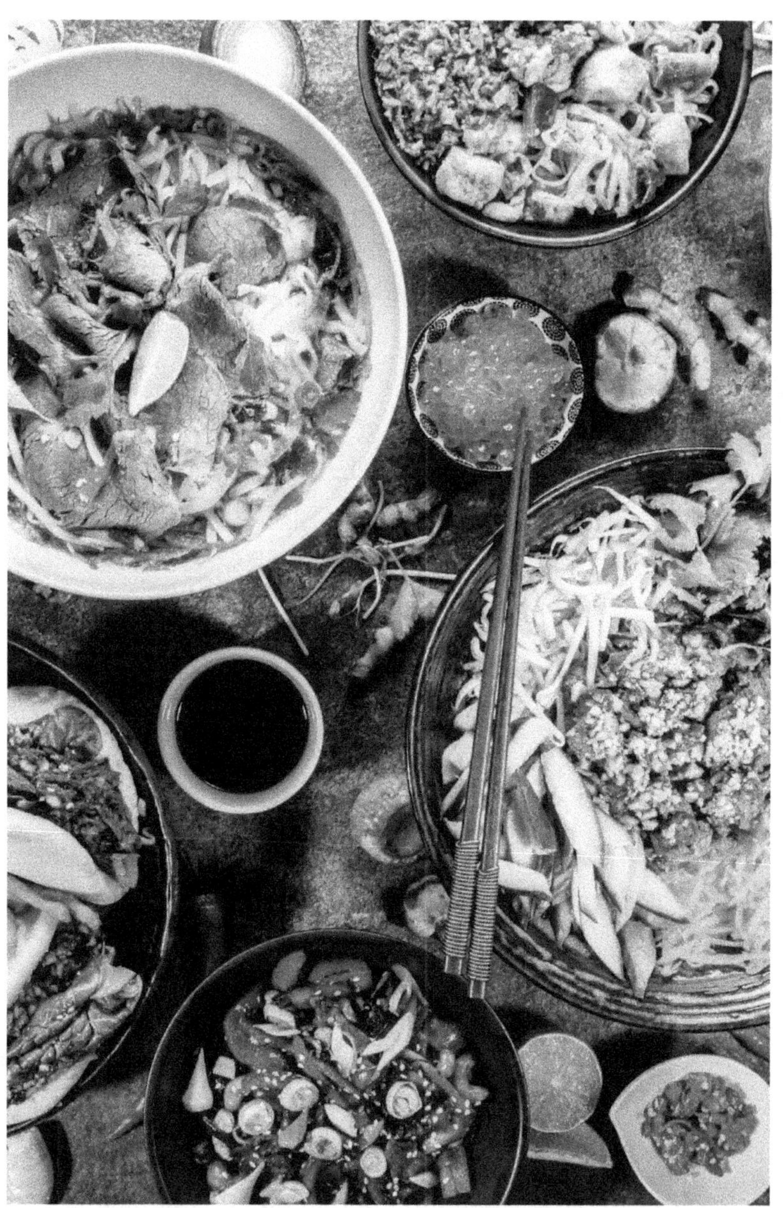

# TABLE OF CONTENTS

# INTRODUCTION

Diabetes and kidney health are closely intertwined aspects of our overall well-being. To truly appreciate the connection between the two, it's essential to delve into the intricate mechanisms at play within our bodies.

Diabetes, in its various forms, affects how our bodies handle glucose, the primary source of energy derived from the food we consume. When diabetes is poorly managed, the excess glucose in the bloodstream can lead to complications that extend beyond blood sugar control. The kidneys, remarkable organs that filter waste and excess substances from our blood, play a pivotal role in this narrative.

These bean-shaped powerhouses, the kidneys, ensure that our internal environment stays balanced. One of their primary functions is regulating fluid and electrolyte levels in our bodies. But in individuals with uncontrolled diabetes, the kidneys can become overworked, leading to kidney damage, or diabetic nephropathy. This condition can ultimately result in kidney failure, underscoring the significance of diabetes management for kidney health.

## The Importance of a Balanced Diet

Now, let's shift our focus to the bedrock of managing both diabetes and kidney health: a balanced diet. Food choices are paramount, as they directly influence blood sugar levels, overall health, and, in the case of individuals with diabetes, the strain on the kidneys.

A balanced diet is one that encompasses a variety of foods from different food groups, providing a spectrum of essential nutrients. For those with diabetes, managing carbohydrate intake is pivotal. Carbohydrates impact blood sugar levels the most, so it's crucial to choose complex carbohydrates that release glucose slowly, such as whole grains, legumes, and vegetables. This promotes stable blood sugar levels, reducing stress on both the pancreas and the kidneys.

Moreover, limiting sodium intake is essential for kidney health. Excess sodium can lead to high blood pressure and fluid retention, both of which are detrimental to kidney function. By choosing low-sodium options and cooking with herbs and spices instead of salt, you can protect your kidneys while enhancing the flavor of your meals.

Protein, a fundamental building block for our bodies, is another critical element in a balanced diet. For individuals with kidney issues, it's important to manage protein intake to reduce the workload on these vital organs. High-quality sources of protein, like lean meats, fish, and plant-based options, are preferred choices.

In summary, the relationship between diabetes and kidney health is a complex one, with diet playing a pivotal role in maintaining their harmonious coexistence. A balanced diet, tailored to individual needs, can help regulate blood sugar levels, support kidney function, and contribute to a healthier, more vibrant life. By understanding this connection and making informed food choices, you can take significant steps towards managing your health and well-being effectively.

# Chapter 1: 30 Day Meal Plan

## Week 1:

Day 1:

- Breakfast: Oatmeal with Fresh Berries
- Lunch: Grilled Chicken Salad
- Dinner: Baked Salmon with Dill Sauce
- Snack: Guacamole with Veggie Sticks
- Dessert: Sugar-Free Berry Parfait

Day 2:

- Breakfast: Scrambled Eggs with Spinach
- Lunch: Lentil and Vegetable Soup
- Dinner: Lemon Herb Chicken
- Snack: Hummus with Whole Wheat Pita
- Dessert: Dark Chocolate-Covered Strawberries

Day 3:

- Breakfast: Greek Yogurt Parfait
- Lunch: Tuna Salad Lettuce Wraps
- Dinner: Eggplant Parmesan

- Snack: Cucumber Slices with Greek Yogurt Dip
- Dessert: Baked Apples with Cinnamon

Day 4:

- Breakfast: Whole Grain Pancakes
- Lunch: Quinoa and Black Bean Bowl
- Dinner: Turkey Meatloaf
- Snack: Deviled Eggs
- Dessert: Chia Seed Chocolate Pudding

Day 5:

- Breakfast: Avocado Toast with Poached Egg
- Lunch: Turkey and Avocado Wrap
- Dinner: Spaghetti Squash with Pesto
- Snack: Mixed Nuts
- Dessert: Almond and Berry Crisp

Day 6:

- Breakfast: Nut Butter and Banana Smoothie
- Lunch: Minestrone Soup
- Dinner: Spinach and Mushroom Stuffed Chicken
- Snack: Caprese Skewers

- Dessert: Frozen Yogurt Popsicles

Day 7:

- Breakfast: Veggie Omelette
- Lunch: Shrimp and Asparagus Stir-Fry
- Dinner: Cauliflower Fried Rice
- Snack: Cottage Cheese with Pineapple
- Dessert: Mango Sorbet

## Week 2:

Day 8:

- Breakfast: Chia Seed Pudding
- Lunch: Chickpea and Spinach Salad
- Dinner: Blackened Tilapia
- Snack: Sliced Apple with Almond Butter
- Dessert: Rice Pudding with Cinnamon

Day 9:

- Breakfast: Quinoa Breakfast Bowl
- Lunch: Teriyaki Salmon with Brown Rice
- Dinner: Grilled Portobello Mushrooms
- Snack: Smoked Salmon Roll-Ups

- Dessert: Poached Pears in Red Wine

Day 10:

- Breakfast: Cottage Cheese and Fruit
- Lunch: Caprese Salad
- Dinner: Pork Tenderloin with Apple Compote
- Snack: Baked Sweet Potato Fries
- Dessert: Pumpkin Pie Smoothie

Day 11:

- Breakfast: Sweet Potato Hash
- Lunch: Black Bean and Corn Tacos
- Dinner: Ratatouille
- Snack: Edamame
- Dessert: Almond Joy Bites

Day 12:

- Breakfast: Breakfast Burrito
- Lunch: Cucumber and Tomato Salad
- Dinner: Zucchini Noodles with Marinara
- Snack: Greek Salad Cups
- Dessert: Lemon Ricotta Cheesecake

Day 13:

- Breakfast: Muesli with Nuts and Seeds
- Lunch: Beef and Vegetable Stir-Fry
- Dinner: Sweet and Sour Tofu
- Snack: Salsa with Baked Tortilla Chips
- Dessert: Peach and Blueberry Cobbler

Day 14:

- Breakfast: Spinach and Feta Quiche
- Lunch: Mediterranean Quinoa Salad
- Dinner: Stuffed Bell Peppers
- Snack: Stuffed Mushrooms
- Dessert: Carrot Cake Bites

## Week 3:

Day 15:

- Breakfast: Oatmeal with Fresh Berries
- Lunch: Grilled Chicken Salad
- Dinner: Baked Salmon with Dill Sauce
- Snack: Guacamole with Veggie Sticks
- Dessert: Sugar-Free Berry Parfait

Day 16:

- Breakfast: Scrambled Eggs with Spinach
- Lunch: Lentil and Vegetable Soup
- Dinner: Lemon Herb Chicken
- Snack: Hummus with Whole Wheat Pita
- Dessert: Dark Chocolate-Covered Strawberries

Day 17:

- Breakfast: Greek Yogurt Parfait
- Lunch: Tuna Salad Lettuce Wraps
- Dinner: Eggplant Parmesan
- Snack: Cucumber Slices with Greek Yogurt Dip
- Dessert: Baked Apples with Cinnamon

Day 18:

- Breakfast: Whole Grain Pancakes
- Lunch: Quinoa and Black Bean Bowl
- Dinner: Turkey Meatloaf
- Snack: Deviled Eggs
- Dessert: Chia Seed Chocolate Pudding

Day 19:

- Breakfast: Avocado Toast with Poached Egg
- Lunch: Turkey and Avocado Wrap
- Dinner: Spaghetti Squash with Pesto
- Snack: Mixed Nuts
- Dessert: Almond and Berry Crisp

Day 20:

- Breakfast: Nut Butter and Banana Smoothie
- Lunch: Minestrone Soup
- Dinner: Spinach and Mushroom Stuffed Chicken
- Snack: Caprese Skewers
- Dessert: Frozen Yogurt Popsicles

Day 21:

- Breakfast: Veggie Omelette
- Lunch: Shrimp and Asparagus Stir-Fry
- Dinner: Cauliflower Fried Rice
- Snack: Cottage Cheese with Pineapple
- Dessert: Mango Sorbet

# Week 4:

Day 22:

- Breakfast: Chia Seed Pudding
- Lunch: Chickpea and Spinach Salad
- Dinner: Blackened Tilapia
- Snack: Sliced Apple with Almond Butter
- Dessert: Rice Pudding with Cinnamon

Day 23:

- Breakfast: Quinoa Breakfast Bowl
- Lunch: Teriyaki Salmon with Brown Rice
- Dinner: Grilled Portobello Mushrooms
- Snack: Smoked Salmon Roll-Ups
- Dessert: Poached Pears in Red Wine

Day 24:

- Breakfast: Cottage Cheese and Fruit
- Lunch: Caprese Salad
- Dinner: Pork Tenderloin with Apple Compote
- Snack: Baked Sweet Potato Fries
- Dessert: Pumpkin Pie Smoothie

Day 25:

- Breakfast: Sweet Potato Hash
- Lunch: Black Bean and Corn Tacos
- Dinner: Ratatouille
- Snack: Edamame
- Dessert: Almond Joy Bites

Day 26:

- Breakfast: Breakfast Burrito
- Lunch: Cucumber and Tomato Salad
- Dinner: Zucchini Noodles with Marinara
- Snack: Greek Salad Cups
- Dessert: Lemon Ricotta Cheesecake

Day 27:

- Breakfast: Muesli with Nuts and Seeds
- Lunch: Beef and Vegetable Stir-Fry
- Dinner: Sweet and Sour Tofu
- Snack: Salsa with Baked Tortilla Chips
- Dessert: Peach and Blueberry Cobbler

Day 28:

- Breakfast: Spinach and Feta Quiche
- Lunch: Mediterranean Quinoa Salad
- Dinner: Stuffed Bell Peppers
- Snack: Stuffed Mushrooms
- Dessert: Carrot Cake Bites

Day 29:

- Breakfast: Oatmeal with Fresh Berries
- Lunch: Grilled Chicken Salad
- Dinner: Baked Salmon with Dill Sauce
- Snack: Guacamole with Veggie Sticks
- Dessert: Sugar-Free Berry Parfait

Day 30:

- Breakfast: Scrambled Eggs with Spinach
- Lunch: Lentil and Vegetable Soup
- Dinner: Lemon Herb Chicken
- Snack: Hummus with Whole Wheat Pita
- Dessert: Dark Chocolate-Covered Strawberries

Congratulations! You've completed a full 30-day meal plan with a diverse range of recipes for breakfast, lunch, dinner, snacks, and dessert. Continue to adjust portion sizes and ingredients as needed to meet your specific dietary requirements and health goals.

# Chapter 2: Breakfast Recipes

Breakfast is a cherished opportunity to fuel your body with a healthy burst of energy, especially if you're managing diabetes and kidney health. In this chapter, you'll discover a treasure trove of wholesome and delicious breakfast recipes that are not only gentle on your health but also tantalizing to your taste buds.

## Oatmeal with Fresh Berries

Ingredients:

- 1/2 cup rolled oats
- 1 cup almond milk
- 1/4 cup fresh berries (strawberries, blueberries, or raspberries)
- 1 tablespoon honey
- 1/4 teaspoon cinnamon

Instructions:

1. In a saucepan, combine rolled oats and almond milk.

2. Cook over medium heat, stirring frequently, until the oats absorb the liquid and achieve a creamy consistency.
3. Transfer the oatmeal to a bowl.
4. Top with fresh berries, drizzle with honey, and sprinkle with cinnamon.
5. Enjoy your wholesome berry-infused oatmeal.

## Scrambled Eggs with Spinach

Ingredients:

- 2 eggs
- 1 cup fresh spinach leaves
- Salt and pepper to taste
- 1 teaspoon olive oil

Instructions:

1. Heat olive oil in a pan over medium heat.
2. Add fresh spinach and sauté until wilted.
3. In a bowl, beat the eggs with salt and pepper.
4. Pour the beaten eggs into the pan with spinach.
5. Cook, stirring gently, until the eggs are scrambled to your liking.

6. Serve your nutrient-packed scrambled eggs with a
   side of spinach.


## Greek Yogurt Parfait

Ingredients:

- 1 cup Greek yogurt
- 1/2 cup granola
- 1/4 cup fresh mixed berries
- 1 tablespoon honey

Instructions:

1. In a glass, start with a layer of Greek yogurt.
2. Add a layer of granola on top.
3. Follow with a layer of fresh mixed berries.
4. Drizzle honey over the berries.
5. Repeat the layers if desired.
6. Savor the delightful medley of flavors and textures
   in your parfait.

# Whole Grain Pancakes

Ingredients:

- 1 cup whole grain pancake mix
- 1 cup almond milk
- 1 egg
- 1/2 teaspoon vanilla extract
- Fresh fruit for topping (e.g., sliced bananas or berries)

Instructions:

1. In a bowl, whisk together pancake mix, almond milk, egg, and vanilla extract until smooth.
2. Heat a non-stick skillet over medium heat and lightly grease it.
3. Pour a ladle of the pancake batter onto the skillet to form a pancake.
4. Cook until bubbles appear on the surface, then flip and cook until golden brown.
5. Serve with fresh fruit as a nutritious topping.

# Avocado Toast with Poached Egg

Ingredients:

- 1 slice whole wheat bread
- 1 ripe avocado
- 1 poached egg
- Salt and pepper to taste
- Red pepper flakes (optional)

Instructions:

1. Toast the whole wheat bread to your desired level of crispiness.
2. Mash the ripe avocado and spread it on the toasted bread.
3. Place the poached egg on top of the avocado.
4. Season with salt, pepper, and a pinch of red pepper flakes if you like some heat.
5. Enjoy the creamy and satisfying avocado toast.

# Nut Butter and Banana Smoothie

Ingredients:

- 1 banana

- 2 tablespoons nut butter (almond, peanut, or your choice)
- 1 cup almond milk
- 1 tablespoon honey
- Ice cubes (optional)

Instructions:

1. In a blender, combine banana, nut butter, almond milk, and honey.
2. Add ice cubes if you want a colder smoothie.
3. Blend until smooth and creamy.
4. Pour into a glass and relish this nutritious and protein-packed smoothie.

## Veggie Omelette

Ingredients:

- 2 eggs
- 1/4 cup diced bell peppers
- 1/4 cup diced tomatoes
- 1/4 cup diced onions
- Salt and pepper to taste
- 1 teaspoon olive oil

Instructions:

1. In a bowl, beat the eggs with salt and pepper.

2. Heat olive oil in a pan over medium heat.

3. Add diced bell peppers, tomatoes, and onions to the pan and sauté until tender.

4. Pour the beaten eggs over the sautéed veggies.

5. Cook until the omelette is set and slightly browned.

6. Fold in half and serve your veggie omelette hot.

## Chia Seed Pudding

Ingredients:

- 2 tablespoons chia seeds
- 1 cup unsweetened almond milk
- 1/2 teaspoon vanilla extract
- Fresh fruit for topping (e.g., sliced strawberries or kiwi)

Instructions:

1. In a container or jar, combine chia seeds, almond milk, and vanilla extract.

2. Stir well and refrigerate overnight or for at least 4 hours.

3. Before serving, top with fresh fruit for a burst of
   flavor.

## Quinoa Breakfast Bowl

Ingredients:

- 1/2 cup cooked quinoa
- 1/4 cup unsweetened Greek yogurt
- 1/4 cup fresh mixed berries
- 1 tablespoon honey
- Nuts or seeds for added crunch (optional)

Instructions:

1. In a bowl, layer cooked quinoa with Greek yogurt.
2. Top with fresh mixed berries and drizzle honey over
   the bowl.
3. Sprinkle with nuts or seeds for extra texture.
4. Relish this nutritious and satisfying breakfast.

## Cottage Cheese and Fruit

Ingredients:

- 1/2 cup low-fat cottage cheese

- 1/2 cup fresh fruit (e.g., pineapple, peaches, or melon)
- A sprinkle of ground cinnamon

Instructions:

1. Spoon the cottage cheese into a bowl.
2. Add fresh fruit on top.
3. Finish with a sprinkle of ground cinnamon for a touch of warmth.
4. Savor the creaminess and sweetness of this simple delight.

## Sweet Potato Hash

Ingredients:

- 1 medium sweet potato, peeled and diced
- 1/4 cup diced red bell pepper
- 1/4 cup diced red onion
- 1/2 teaspoon smoked paprika
- 1 teaspoon olive oil

Instructions:

1. Heat olive oil in a skillet over medium heat.

2. Add diced sweet potato, bell pepper, and onion to the skillet.

3. Sprinkle with smoked paprika and cook until sweet potatoes are tender and slightly crispy.

4. Serve this savory and colorful hash.

## Breakfast Burrito

Ingredients:

- 2 scrambled eggs
- 1 whole wheat tortilla
- 1/4 cup black beans
- 1/4 cup diced tomatoes
- Salsa for added flavor

Instructions:

1. Place the scrambled eggs, black beans, and diced tomatoes on a whole wheat tortilla.

2. Add salsa for an extra kick.

3. Roll it up into a burrito and enjoy a hearty breakfast on the go.

## Muesli with Nuts and Seeds

Ingredients:

- 1/2 cup muesli cereal
- 1/4 cup chopped nuts (e.g., almonds or walnuts)
- 2 tablespoons mixed seeds (e.g., chia, flax, or pumpkin seeds)
- 1/2 cup unsweetened almond milk

Instructions:

1. Combine muesli cereal, chopped nuts, and mixed seeds in a bowl.
2. Pour almond milk over the mixture.
3. Let it sit for a few minutes to soften, and then dig in.

## Spinach and Feta Quiche

Ingredients:

- 1 pre-made whole wheat pie crust
- 4 eggs
- 1 cup fresh spinach, chopped
- 1/2 cup crumbled feta cheese
- Salt and pepper to taste

Instructions:

1. Preheat the oven according to the pie crust instructions.
2. In a bowl, whisk together eggs, chopped spinach, feta cheese, salt, and pepper.
3. Pour the mixture into the pie crust.
4. Bake as per the pie crust instructions until the quiche is set and golden brown.
5. Slice and serve this savory quiche.

## Veggie Breakfast Casserole

Ingredients:

- 6 eggs
- 1 cup diced mixed vegetables (e.g., bell peppers, zucchini, and onions)
- 1 cup shredded low-fat cheese
- Salt and pepper to taste

Instructions:

1. Preheat the oven to 350°F (175°C).
2. In a baking dish, layer the diced vegetables.

3. In a bowl, beat the eggs and season with salt and pepper.

4. Pour the beaten eggs over the vegetables.

5. Sprinkle the shredded cheese on top.

6. Bake for about 30 minutes or until the casserole is set and the cheese is bubbly.

7. Cut into squares and enjoy this satisfying breakfast casserole.

# Chapter 3: Lunch Recipes

In this chapter, we're diving into the world of delicious and nutritious lunch options that are not only satisfying but also perfect for those looking after their diabetes and kidney health. These recipes strike a balance between flavor and health, ensuring that your midday meal is both enjoyable and beneficial.

## Grilled Chicken Salad

Ingredients:

- 2 boneless, skinless chicken breasts
- 4 cups mixed greens
- 1 cup cherry tomatoes, halved
- 1/2 cucumber, sliced
- 1/4 red onion, thinly sliced
- Balsamic vinaigrette dressing
- Salt and pepper to taste

Instructions:

1. Season the chicken breasts with salt and pepper, then grill until cooked through.
2. Slice the grilled chicken into strips.
3. Toss mixed greens, cherry tomatoes, cucumber, and red onion together in a large bowl.
4. Top the salad with grilled chicken and drizzle with balsamic vinaigrette.

## Lentil and Vegetable Soup

Ingredients:

- 1 cup green or brown lentils
- 1 onion, chopped
- 2 carrots, diced
- 2 celery stalks, chopped
- 4 cups vegetable broth
- 1 can diced tomatoes
- 1 tsp cumin
- 1 tsp coriander
- Salt and pepper to taste

Instructions:

1.  Sauté the onion, carrots, and celery in a large pot until they start to soften.

2.  Add the lentils, vegetable broth, diced tomatoes, and spices.

3.  Simmer for 30-40 minutes until the lentils are tender.

4.  Season with salt and pepper to taste.

## Tuna Salad Lettuce Wraps

Ingredients:

- 2 cans of tuna in water, drained
- 1/4 cup Greek yogurt
- 1/4 cup diced red onion
- 1/4 cup diced celery
- 1 tbsp lemon juice
- Salt and pepper to taste
- Large lettuce leaves

Instructions:

1.  In a bowl, mix the tuna, Greek yogurt, red onion, celery, and lemon juice.

2.  Season with salt and pepper.

3. Spoon the tuna salad into large lettuce leaves and wrap them up.

## Quinoa and Black Bean Bowl

Ingredients:

- 1 cup cooked quinoa
- 1 can black beans, drained and rinsed
- 1 cup corn kernels
- 1 red bell pepper, diced
- 1/4 cup cilantro, chopped
- Lime vinaigrette dressing

Instructions:

1. In a bowl, combine quinoa, black beans, corn, red bell pepper, and cilantro.
2. Drizzle with lime vinaigrette dressing and toss to combine.

## Turkey and Avocado Wrap

Ingredients:

- 4 whole wheat tortillas

- 1/2 pound thinly sliced turkey breast
- 1 avocado, sliced
- 1 cup spinach leaves
- 1/4 cup Greek yogurt
- 1 tsp Dijon mustard

Instructions:

1. Lay out tortillas and spread Greek yogurt and Dijon mustard.
2. Layer turkey, avocado, and spinach on each tortilla.
3. Roll them up and slice in half.

## Minestrone Soup

Ingredients:

- 1 cup diced onion
- 1 cup chopped carrots
- 1 cup chopped celery
- 2 cloves garlic, minced
- 1 can kidney beans, drained and rinsed
- 1 can diced tomatoes
- 6 cups vegetable broth
- 1 cup small pasta (like elbow macaroni)

- 1 tsp Italian seasoning
- Salt and pepper to taste

Instructions:

1. In a large pot, sauté the onion, carrots, celery, and garlic until tender.
2. Add kidney beans, diced tomatoes, vegetable broth, pasta, and Italian seasoning.
3. Simmer until the pasta is cooked.
4. Season with salt and pepper.

## Shrimp and Asparagus Stir-Fry

Ingredients:

- 1 pound large shrimp, peeled and deveined
- 1 bunch asparagus, trimmed and cut into pieces
- 1 red bell pepper, sliced
- 2 cloves garlic, minced
- 2 tbsp low-sodium soy sauce
- 1 tsp ginger, grated
- 1 tsp honey
- 1 tbsp olive oil

Instructions:

1. Heat olive oil in a wok or large pan.

2. Add shrimp and stir-fry until pink.

3. Add asparagus, red bell pepper, garlic, and ginger. Stir-fry for a few more minutes.

4. In a small bowl, mix soy sauce and honey. Pour over the stir-fry and toss to combine.

## Chickpea and Spinach Salad

Ingredients:

- 2 cups cooked chickpeas
- 2 cups fresh spinach leaves
- 1/4 cup feta cheese, crumbled
- 1/4 cup red onion, thinly sliced
- Balsamic vinaigrette dressing
- Salt and pepper to taste

Instructions:

1. In a large bowl, combine chickpeas, spinach, feta cheese, and red onion.

2. Drizzle with balsamic vinaigrette and season with salt and pepper.

# Teriyaki Salmon with Brown Rice

Ingredients:

- 4 salmon fillets
- 1/4 cup low-sodium teriyaki sauce
- 2 cups cooked brown rice
- 1 cup steamed broccoli

Instructions:

1. Marinate salmon in teriyaki sauce for about 15 minutes.
2. Grill or bake the salmon until it flakes easily.
3. Serve over brown rice and steamed broccoli.

# Caprese Salad

Ingredients:

- 4 ripe tomatoes, sliced
- 1 cup fresh mozzarella cheese, sliced
- 1/4 cup fresh basil leaves
- Balsamic glaze
- Olive oil
- Salt and pepper to taste

Instructions:

1. Arrange tomato and mozzarella slices on a platter.

2. Tuck basil leaves between the slices.

3. Drizzle with olive oil and balsamic glaze. Season with salt and pepper.

## Black Bean and Corn Tacos

Ingredients:

- 1 can black beans, drained and rinsed
- 1 cup corn kernels
- 1 red bell pepper, diced
- 1/2 tsp chili powder
- 1/2 tsp cumin
- 8 small whole wheat tortillas
- Toppings: salsa, Greek yogurt, shredded lettuce

Instructions:

1. In a pan, combine black beans, corn, red bell pepper, chili powder, and cumin. Heat until warm.

2. Warm the tortillas in the oven or on a griddle.

3. Fill the tortillas with the black bean mixture and your choice of toppings.

# Cucumber and Tomato Salad

Ingredients:

- 2 cucumbers, sliced
- 2 cups cherry tomatoes, halved
- 1/4 red onion, thinly sliced
- 1/4 cup fresh dill, chopped
- Feta cheese (optional)
- Lemon vinaigrette dressing
- Salt and pepper to taste

Instructions:

1. In a large bowl, combine cucumbers, cherry tomatoes, red onion, and dill.
2. If desired, sprinkle with crumbled feta cheese.
3. Drizzle with lemon vinaigrette and season with salt and pepper.

# Beef and Vegetable Stir-Fry

Ingredients:

- 1 pound lean beef, thinly sliced
- 2 cups broccoli florets

- 1 red bell pepper, sliced

- 1 cup snap peas

- 2 cloves garlic, minced

- 2 tbsp low-sodium soy sauce

- 1 tsp sesame oil

- 1 tsp ginger, grated

Instructions:

1. In a wok or large pan, stir-fry beef until browned. Remove and set aside.

2. In the same pan, stir-fry broccoli, red bell pepper, snap peas, and garlic.

3. Return beef to the pan and add soy sauce, sesame oil, and ginger. Stir until heated through.

## Mediterranean Quinoa Salad

Ingredients:

- 1 cup cooked quinoa

- 1 cup cherry tomatoes, halved

- 1 cucumber, diced

- 1/4 cup Kalamata olives, pitted and sliced

- 1/4 cup feta cheese, crumbled

- Red wine vinaigrette dressing

- Fresh parsley for garnish

- Salt and pepper to taste

Instructions:

1. In a bowl, combine quinoa, cherry tomatoes, cucumber, Kalamata olives, and feta cheese.

2. Drizzle with red wine vinaigrette and garnish with fresh parsley. Season with salt and pepper.

## Mushroom and Barley Soup

Ingredients:

- 1 cup pearl barley

- 8 cups vegetable broth

- 1 cup mushrooms, sliced

- 1 cup carrots, diced

- 1 cup celery, chopped

- 1 onion, chopped

- 2 cloves garlic, minced

- 1 tsp thyme

- Salt and pepper to taste

Instructions:

1.  In a large pot, combine barley and vegetable broth. Bring to a boil, then reduce heat and simmer for 20 minutes.

2.  In a separate pan, sauté mushrooms, carrots, celery, onion, and garlic.

3.  Add the sautéed vegetables to the pot with the barley.

4.  Season with thyme, salt, and pepper. Simmer until barley is tender.

# Chapter 4: Dinner Recipes

When it comes to satisfying dinners that cater to both diabetes and kidney health, this chapter presents a delightful array of recipes that not only tantalize your taste buds but also support your well-being. From succulent salmon to flavorful tofu, these recipes are thoughtfully crafted to provide a variety of options for your evening meals.

## Baked Salmon with Dill Sauce

Ingredients:

- 4 salmon fillets
- 2 tablespoons olive oil
- 1 tablespoon lemon juice
- 1 teaspoon dried dill
- Salt and pepper to taste

Instructions:

1. Preheat your oven to 375°F (190°C).
2. Place the salmon fillets on a baking sheet.
3. Drizzle them with olive oil and lemon juice.

4. Sprinkle with dried dill, salt, and pepper.

5. Bake for 15-20 minutes or until the salmon flakes easily with a fork.

6. Serve with a dollop of dill sauce.

## Lemon Herb Chicken

Ingredients:

- 4 boneless, skinless chicken breasts
- 2 tablespoons olive oil
- 1 lemon, juiced and zested
- 2 cloves garlic, minced
- 1 teaspoon dried basil
- Salt and pepper to taste

Instructions:

1. In a bowl, mix the olive oil, lemon juice, lemon zest, minced garlic, dried basil, salt, and pepper.

2. Marinate the chicken breasts in this mixture for 30 minutes.

3. Grill or pan-sear the chicken until fully cooked, about 6-7 minutes per side.

4. Serve with a garnish of fresh herbs.

# Eggplant Parmesan

Ingredients:

- 2 large eggplants, sliced
- 2 cups marinara sauce
- 1 cup part-skim mozzarella cheese, grated
- 1/2 cup Parmesan cheese, grated
- 1/4 cup breadcrumbs
- Fresh basil leaves for garnish

Instructions:

1. Preheat your oven to 375°F (190°C).
2. Lightly salt eggplant slices and let them sit for 30 minutes to remove excess moisture.
3. Rinse and pat dry, then coat each slice with breadcrumbs.
4. Layer eggplant, marinara sauce, and cheeses in a baking dish.
5. Repeat the layers and top with mozzarella and Parmesan.
6. Bake for 30-35 minutes or until bubbly and golden.
7. Garnish with fresh basil leaves.

# Turkey Meatloaf

Ingredients:

- 1 pound ground turkey
- 1/2 cup rolled oats
- 1/2 cup low-sodium tomato sauce
- 1/2 cup finely chopped onion
- 1/4 cup finely chopped green bell pepper
- 1/4 cup finely chopped celery
- 2 cloves garlic, minced
- 1 egg
- 1 teaspoon dried thyme
- Salt and pepper to taste

Instructions:

1. Preheat your oven to 375°F (190°C).
2. In a bowl, combine all the ingredients and mix well.
3. Shape the mixture into a loaf and place it in a baking dish.
4. Bake for 45-50 minutes or until the internal temperature reaches 165°F (74°C).

# Spaghetti Squash with Pesto

Ingredients:

- 1 spaghetti squash
- 1/2 cup basil pesto
- Cherry tomatoes, halved
- Grated Parmesan cheese
- Fresh basil leaves for garnish

Instructions:

1. Preheat your oven to 375°F (190°C).
2. Cut the spaghetti squash in half lengthwise and scoop out the seeds.
3. Place the halves cut-side down on a baking sheet and roast for 40-45 minutes.
4. Scrape the cooked squash into "noodles" with a fork.
5. Toss with pesto, cherry tomatoes, and top with grated Parmesan and fresh basil leaves.

# Spinach and Mushroom Stuffed Chicken

Ingredients:

- 4 boneless, skinless chicken breasts
- 1 cup fresh spinach
- 1 cup mushrooms, chopped
- 1/2 cup low-fat cream cheese
- 2 cloves garlic, minced
- Salt and pepper to taste

Instructions:

1. Preheat your oven to 375°F (190°C).
2. In a skillet, sauté the mushrooms and garlic until tender.
3. Add spinach and cook until wilted.
4. Stir in cream cheese and season with salt and pepper.
5. Cut a pocket into each chicken breast, then stuff with the spinach and mushroom mixture.
6. Bake for 25-30 minutes or until chicken is cooked through.

# Cauliflower Fried Rice

Ingredients:

- 1 head of cauliflower, grated
- 2 cups mixed vegetables (peas, carrots, bell peppers)
- 2 cloves garlic, minced
- 2 tablespoons low-sodium soy sauce
- 1 tablespoon sesame oil
- 2 eggs, beaten
- Green onions for garnish

Instructions:

1. In a large pan, heat sesame oil and sauté the garlic.
2. Add the mixed vegetables and cook until tender.
3. Push the vegetables to one side and scramble the eggs on the other side of the pan.
4. Stir in the cauliflower rice and soy sauce. Cook until heated through.
5. Garnish with chopped green onions.

## Blackened Tilapia

Ingredients:

- 4 tilapia fillets
- 2 teaspoons paprika
- 1 teaspoon dried thyme
- 1 teaspoon garlic powder
- 1/2 teaspoon cayenne pepper
- 1/2 teaspoon onion powder
- Salt and pepper to taste
- Olive oil for cooking

Instructions:

1. In a bowl, combine paprika, thyme, garlic powder, cayenne pepper, onion powder, salt, and pepper.
2. Coat each tilapia fillet with the spice mixture.
3. Heat olive oil in a pan and cook the fillets for 3-4 minutes per side or until flaky.

## Grilled Portobello Mushrooms

Ingredients:

- 4 large Portobello mushrooms

- 2 tablespoons balsamic vinegar

- 2 tablespoons olive oil

- 2 cloves garlic, minced

- Salt and pepper to taste

- Fresh parsley for garnish

Instructions:

1. In a bowl, mix balsamic vinegar, olive oil, minced garlic, salt, and pepper.
2. Brush the Portobello mushrooms with the mixture.
3. Grill for 4-5 minutes per side.
4. Garnish with fresh parsley.

## Pork Tenderloin with Apple Compote

Ingredients:

- 1 pork tenderloin

- 2 apples, peeled, cored, and chopped

- 1/4 cup apple cider vinegar

- 1/4 cup water

- 2 tablespoons honey

- 1 teaspoon ground cinnamon
- Salt and pepper to taste

Instructions:

1. Preheat your oven to 375°F (190°C).
2. Season the pork tenderloin with salt and pepper.
3. Sear it in a hot, oven-safe pan until browned on all sides.
4. In a separate pan, cook apples, apple cider vinegar, water, honey, and cinnamon until apples are tender and compote forms.
5. Pour the compote over the pork and roast for 20-25 minutes or until fully cooked.

## Ratatouille

Ingredients:

- 1 eggplant, sliced
- 2 zucchinis, sliced
- 2 bell peppers, sliced
- 4 tomatoes, sliced
- 2 onions, sliced
- 2 cloves garlic, minced

- 1/4 cup olive oil

- 1 teaspoon dried thyme

- Salt and pepper to taste

Instructions:

1. Preheat your oven to 375°F (190°C).

2. Layer the sliced vegetables in a baking dish.

3. Drizzle with olive oil and sprinkle with thyme, salt, and pepper.

4. Bake for 40-45 minutes or until vegetables are tender.

## Zucchini Noodles with Marinara

Ingredients:

- 4 zucchinis, spiralized into noodles

- 2 cups marinara sauce

- 1/4 cup grated Parmesan cheese

- Fresh basil leaves for garnish

Instructions:

1. In a large pan, heat the marinara sauce.

2. Add the zucchini noodles and cook until tender, about 3-4 minutes.

3. Serve with grated Parmesan cheese and fresh basil leaves.

## Beef and Broccoli Stir-Fry

Ingredients:

- 1 pound lean beef, thinly sliced
- 2 cups broccoli florets
- 2 cloves garlic, minced
- 1/4 cup low-sodium soy sauce
- 1 tablespoon honey
- 1 tablespoon cornstarch
- Sesame seeds for garnish

Instructions:

1. In a bowl, mix soy sauce, honey, and cornstarch.
2. In a large pan, stir-fry beef until browned. Remove from the pan.
3. Add garlic and broccoli to the pan and stir-fry until tender.
4. Return the beef to the pan and pour the sauce over it.

5. Cook until the sauce thickens.

6. Garnish with sesame seeds.

## Sweet and Sour Tofu

Ingredients:

- 1 block extra-firm tofu, cubed
- 1/2 cup pineapple chunks
- 1/4 cup low-sodium soy sauce
- 2 tablespoons rice vinegar
- 2 tablespoons honey
- 1/2 teaspoon ginger, minced
- 1/2 teaspoon garlic, minced
- 1 bell pepper, sliced

Instructions:

1. In a bowl, mix soy sauce, rice vinegar, honey, ginger, and garlic.
2. Heat a pan, add tofu, and cook until golden.
3. Add bell pepper and pineapple chunks to the pan.
4. Pour the sauce over the tofu and vegetables, and cook until heated through.

## Stuffed Bell Peppers

Ingredients:

- 4 bell peppers, tops removed and seeds removed
- 1 cup cooked quinoa
- 1 cup lean ground beef or turkey
- 1/2 cup black beans, drained and rinsed
- 1/2 cup corn
- 1 cup low-sodium tomato sauce
- 1 teaspoon chili powder
- 1/2 teaspoon cumin
- Salt and pepper to taste

Instructions:

1. Preheat your oven to 375°F (190°C).
2. In a pan, brown the ground meat and drain excess fat.
3. Mix meat, cooked quinoa, black beans, corn, tomato sauce, chili powder, cumin, salt, and pepper.
4. Stuff the bell peppers with the mixture.
5. Bake for 25-30 minutes or until peppers are tender.

# Chapter 5: Snacks and Appetizers

This chapter is dedicated to a delightful assortment of snacks and appetizers that not only satisfy your taste buds but also support your diabetes and kidney health goals. From classic favorites to inventive bites, these recipes provide a balance of flavor and nutrition.

## Guacamole with Veggie Sticks

Ingredients:

- 2 ripe avocados
- 1 small red onion, finely diced
- 1-2 cloves garlic, minced
- 2 ripe tomatoes, diced
- 1 lime, juiced
- 1/2 teaspoon salt
- 1/4 teaspoon black pepper
- Assorted vegetable sticks (carrots, celery, bell peppers) for dipping

Instructions:

1. Cut the avocados in half, remove the pit, and scoop the flesh into a bowl.

2. Mash the avocados with a fork or potato masher.

3. Add diced onion, minced garlic, diced tomatoes, lime juice, salt, and pepper. Mix well.

4. Serve with vegetable sticks for dipping.

## Hummus with Whole Wheat Pita

Ingredients:

- 1 can (15 oz) chickpeas, drained and rinsed
- 2 cloves garlic, minced
- 3 tablespoons tahini
- 3 tablespoons lemon juice
- 2 tablespoons olive oil
- 1/2 teaspoon ground cumin
- Salt and pepper to taste
- Whole wheat pita bread, cut into triangles

Instructions:

1.  In a food processor, combine chickpeas, minced garlic, tahini, lemon juice, olive oil, ground cumin, salt, and pepper.

2.  Blend until smooth, adding a little water if needed for desired consistency.

3.  Serve with whole wheat pita triangles.

## Cucumber Slices with Greek Yogurt Dip

Ingredients:

- 1 cucumber, thinly sliced
- 1 cup Greek yogurt
- 1 tablespoon fresh dill, chopped
- 1 teaspoon lemon juice
- Salt and pepper to taste

Instructions:

1.  In a bowl, mix Greek yogurt, fresh dill, lemon juice, salt, and pepper.

2.  Serve cucumber slices with the yogurt dip.

# Deviled Eggs

Ingredients:

- 6 hard-boiled eggs, peeled
- 3 tablespoons Greek yogurt
- 1 teaspoon Dijon mustard
- 1/2 teaspoon paprika
- Chopped chives for garnish

Instructions:

1. Cut hard-boiled eggs in half lengthwise. Remove yolks and place them in a bowl.
2. Mash the yolks and mix with Greek yogurt, Dijon mustard, and paprika.
3. Fill the egg white halves with the yolk mixture.
4. Garnish with chopped chives.

# Mixed Nuts

Ingredients:

- A mixture of unsalted almonds, walnuts, cashews, and pistachios

Instructions:

1.  Simply mix the assorted unsalted nuts together.

2.  Serve as a heart-healthy snack.

## Caprese Skewers

Ingredients:

- Cherry tomatoes

- Fresh mozzarella balls

- Fresh basil leaves

- Balsamic glaze

Instructions:

1.  Thread cherry tomatoes, mozzarella balls, and fresh basil leaves onto skewers.

2.  Drizzle with balsamic glaze for extra flavor.

## Cottage Cheese with Pineapple

Ingredients:

- 1 cup low-fat cottage cheese

- 1/2 cup diced fresh pineapple

Instructions:

1. Serve a scoop of low-fat cottage cheese topped with diced pineapple.

## Sliced Apple with Almond Butter

Ingredients:

- Sliced apples
- Almond butter

Instructions:

1. Dip apple slices in almond butter for a satisfying and nutritious snack.

## Smoked Salmon Roll-Ups

Ingredients:

- Smoked salmon slices
- Cream cheese
- Fresh dill

Instructions:

1. Spread a thin layer of cream cheese on each smoked salmon slice.
2. Place a sprig of fresh dill on top.
3. Roll up the salmon slices and secure with toothpicks.

## Baked Sweet Potato Fries

Ingredients:

- Sweet potatoes, cut into fries
- Olive oil
- Salt and pepper
- Paprika (optional)

Instructions:

1. Toss sweet potato fries with olive oil, salt, pepper, and paprika.
2. Bake in the oven until crispy.

## Edamame

Ingredients:

- Frozen edamame

- Sea salt

Instructions:

1. Boil or steam edamame until tender.

2. Sprinkle with sea salt and serve.

## Greek Salad Cups

Ingredients:

- Mini phyllo cups

- Cucumber, diced

- Cherry tomatoes, halved

- Feta cheese, crumbled

- Kalamata olives, pitted and chopped

- Fresh oregano leaves

- Olive oil and red wine vinegar for dressing

Instructions:

1. In each phyllo cup, place cucumber, cherry tomato halves, feta cheese, olives, and fresh oregano.

2. Drizzle with a mixture of olive oil and red wine vinegar.

## Salsa with Baked Tortilla Chips

Ingredients:

- Homemade or store-bought salsa
- Baked whole wheat tortilla chips

Instructions:

1. Serve salsa with whole wheat tortilla chips for a crispy, guilt-free snack.

## Stuffed Mushrooms

Ingredients:

- Large mushroom caps
- Spinach and feta stuffing (available in stores)

Instructions:

1. Fill mushroom caps with spinach and feta stuffing.
2. Bake until mushrooms are tender.

## Roasted Red Pepper and Walnut Dip

Ingredients:

- 2 red bell peppers

- 1/2 cup walnuts
- 1 clove garlic
- 1 tablespoon olive oil
- Lemon juice to taste
- Salt and pepper

Instructions:

1. Roast red bell peppers until the skin is charred, then peel and remove the seeds.
2. Blend roasted red peppers, walnuts, garlic, olive oil, lemon juice, salt, and pepper in a food processor until smooth.

# Chapter 6: Desserts

Indulging in delicious desserts is still possible while maintaining your diabetes and kidney health goals. These dessert recipes are not only satisfying but also mindful of your dietary needs. So, let's dive into the world of guilt-free sweetness.

## Sugar-Free Berry Parfait

Ingredients:

- 1 cup of mixed berries (strawberries, blueberries, raspberries)
- 1 cup of sugar-free Greek yogurt
- 2 tablespoons of chopped nuts (almonds or walnuts)
- 1 teaspoon of honey (optional)

Instructions:

1. In a glass, layer a portion of mixed berries at the bottom.
2. Add a layer of sugar-free Greek yogurt on top.

3. Repeat the process, creating beautiful layers of berries and yogurt.

4. Sprinkle chopped nuts on the final layer.

5. Drizzle a bit of honey if desired.

## Dark Chocolate-Covered Strawberries

Ingredients:

- 12 fresh strawberries
- 3 ounces of dark chocolate (at least 70% cocoa)

Instructions:

1. Wash and dry the strawberries thoroughly.

2. Melt the dark chocolate in a microwave or on a double boiler.

3. Dip each strawberry into the melted chocolate, covering them halfway.

4. Place them on a parchment-lined tray.

5. Let them cool until the chocolate hardens.

# Baked Apples with Cinnamon

Ingredients:

- 4 apples (Granny Smith or Gala)
- 2 tablespoons of cinnamon
- 2 tablespoons of chopped nuts (walnuts or pecans)
- 1 tablespoon of sugar substitute

Instructions:

1. Preheat your oven to 350°F (175°C).
2. Core the apples and cut a small slice off the bottom to make them stand.
3. Mix cinnamon, chopped nuts, and sugar substitute in a bowl.
4. Stuff each apple with the mixture.
5. Place the apples in a baking dish and bake for about 30 minutes or until they are soft and tender.

# Chia Seed Chocolate Pudding

Ingredients:

- 1/4 cup of chia seeds
- 1 cup of unsweetened almond milk

- 2 tablespoons of cocoa powder

- 1 tablespoon of sugar substitute

- 1/2 teaspoon of vanilla extract

Instructions:

1. In a bowl, combine chia seeds, almond milk, cocoa powder, sugar substitute, and vanilla extract.
2. Mix well and refrigerate for a few hours or overnight.
3. Stir the mixture before serving.
4. Top with fresh berries or a dollop of whipped cream (sugar-free).

## Almond and Berry Crisp

Ingredients:

- 2 cups of mixed berries (strawberries, blueberries, raspberries)

- 1/2 cup of almond flour

- 1/4 cup of chopped almonds

- 2 tablespoons of sugar substitute

- 2 tablespoons of melted coconut oil

Instructions:

1.  Preheat your oven to 350°F (175°C).

2.  In a mixing bowl, combine mixed berries with sugar substitute.

3.  In a separate bowl, mix almond flour, chopped almonds, and melted coconut oil until crumbly.

4.  Place the berries in a baking dish and sprinkle the almond mixture on top.

5.  Bake for about 20-25 minutes or until the topping is golden and the berries are bubbling.

## Frozen Yogurt Popsicles

Ingredients:

- 2 cups of sugar-free yogurt (Greek or regular)
- 1 cup of mixed berries
- 1 tablespoon of honey (optional)

Instructions:

1.  Mix sugar-free yogurt and mixed berries in a blender until smooth.

2.  Add honey if you prefer a sweeter taste.

3.  Pour the mixture into popsicle molds.

4. Insert popsicle sticks and freeze until solid (usually about 4 hours).

## Mango Sorbet

Ingredients:

- 2 cups of frozen mango chunks
- 1/4 cup of unsweetened almond milk
- 1 tablespoon of lime juice
- 1 tablespoon of sugar substitute

Instructions:

1. Place frozen mango, almond milk, lime juice, and sugar substitute in a blender.
2. Blend until smooth.
3. Transfer the mixture to a container and freeze for a couple of hours until it reaches a sorbet-like consistency.

## Rice Pudding with Cinnamon

Ingredients:

- 1 cup of cooked brown rice

- 2 cups of unsweetened almond milk
- 2 tablespoons of sugar substitute
- 1/2 teaspoon of vanilla extract
- 1/2 teaspoon of ground cinnamon

Instructions:

1.  In a saucepan, combine cooked brown rice, almond milk, sugar substitute, vanilla extract, and ground cinnamon.
2.  Cook over low heat, stirring occasionally, until it thickens (about 20 minutes).
3.  Remove from heat and let it cool.
4.  Serve chilled with a sprinkle of cinnamon on top.

## Poached Pears in Red Wine

Ingredients:

- 4 ripe pears
- 2 cups of red wine (choose a variety low in sugar)
- 1/4 cup of sugar substitute
- 1 cinnamon stick

Instructions:

1.  Peel the pears, leaving the stem intact.

2.  In a saucepan, combine red wine, sugar substitute, and a cinnamon stick.

3.  Add the pears and simmer for about 20 minutes or until they are tender.

4.  Remove from heat and let them cool in the liquid.

## Pumpkin Pie Smoothie

Ingredients:

- 1/2 cup canned pumpkin puree (unsweetened)
- 1/2 banana
- 1 cup unsweetened almond milk
- 1/2 teaspoon pumpkin pie spice
- 1 tablespoon sugar substitute
- Ice cubes (optional)

Instructions:

1.  Blend canned pumpkin, banana, almond milk, pumpkin pie spice, and sugar substitute until smooth.

2.  Add ice cubes for a colder texture, if desired.

3. Serve in a glass and sprinkle a dash of pumpkin pie spice on top.


## Almond Joy Bites

Ingredients:

- 1/2 cup unsweetened shredded coconut
- 1/4 cup almond flour
- 2 tablespoons sugar substitute
- 2 tablespoons coconut oil (melted)
- 2 tablespoons unsweetened dark cocoa powder
- 1/2 teaspoon almond extract

Instructions:

1. In a bowl, combine shredded coconut, almond flour, sugar substitute, melted coconut oil, cocoa powder, and almond extract.
2. Mix until a dough forms.
3. Roll the mixture into small bite-sized balls.
4. Chill in the refrigerator until they firm up.

## Lemon Ricotta Cheesecake

Ingredients:

- 1 cup ricotta cheese (low-fat)
- 1/4 cup lemon juice
- 2 tablespoons sugar substitute
- 1 teaspoon lemon zest
- 1/2 teaspoon vanilla extract
- 2 eggs

Instructions:

1. Preheat your oven to 325°F (160°C).
2. In a mixing bowl, blend ricotta cheese, lemon juice, sugar substitute, lemon zest, and vanilla extract.
3. Add eggs one at a time and mix until smooth.
4. Pour the mixture into a greased baking dish and bake for about 25-30 minutes or until set.
5. Let it cool and refrigerate before serving.

## Peach and Blueberry Cobbler

Ingredients:

- 2 cups of sliced peaches (fresh or frozen)

- 1 cup of fresh blueberries
- 1 cup almond flour
- 2 tablespoons sugar substitute
- 1/4 cup unsweetened almond milk
- 1 teaspoon vanilla extract

Instructions:

1. Preheat your oven to 350°F (175°C).
2. In a baking dish, combine sliced peaches and blueberries.
3. In a separate bowl, mix almond flour, sugar substitute, almond milk, and vanilla extract.
4. Spread the mixture over the fruit.
5. Bake for about 30-35 minutes or until the topping is golden.

## Carrot Cake Bites

Ingredients:

- 1 cup grated carrots
- 1/2 cup almond flour
- 2 tablespoons sugar substitute
- 1/2 teaspoon ground cinnamon

- 1/4 cup unsweetened shredded coconut

Instructions:

1. In a bowl, combine grated carrots, almond flour, sugar substitute, ground cinnamon, and shredded coconut.
2. Roll the mixture into small bite-sized balls.
3. Chill in the refrigerator for an hour.

## Avocado Chocolate Mousse

Ingredients:

- 2 ripe avocados
- 1/4 cup unsweetened cocoa powder
- 1/4 cup sugar substitute
- 1/4 cup unsweetened almond milk
- 1 teaspoon vanilla extract

Instructions:

1. Blend avocados, cocoa powder, sugar substitute, almond milk, and vanilla extract until creamy.
2. Refrigerate for a few hours before serving.

# Chapter 7: Smoothies

In this chapter, we've curated unique and nutritious smoothie recipes that cater to both your taste buds and your health. From refreshing tropical flavors to energizing green detox options, these smoothies are designed to be both satisfying and good for you. Let's dive into the world of wholesome, rejuvenating smoothies.

## Green Detox Smoothie

Ingredients:

- 1 cup spinach leaves
- 1/2 cucumber, peeled and chopped
- 1/2 banana
- 1/2 green apple, cored and sliced
- 1 cup water
- 1/2 lemon, juiced
- Ice cubes (optional)

Instructions:

1. Add spinach, cucumber, banana, green apple, and water to a blender.
2. Squeeze in the lemon juice and add ice cubes if desired.
3. Blend until smooth and serve.

## Berry Blast Smoothie

Ingredients:

- 1 cup mixed berries (strawberries, blueberries, raspberries)
- 1/2 cup plain Greek yogurt
- 1/2 cup almond milk
- 1 tablespoon honey (optional)
- Ice cubes (optional)

Instructions:

1. Combine mixed berries, Greek yogurt, almond milk, and honey in a blender.
2. Add ice cubes for a colder texture.
3. Blend until the mixture is smooth and creamy. Enjoy!

# Tropical Paradise Smoothie

Ingredients:

- 1/2 cup pineapple chunks
- 1/2 banana
- 1/2 cup mango chunks
- 1/2 cup coconut milk
- 1/2 cup orange juice
- Ice cubes (optional)

Instructions:

1. Place pineapple, banana, mango, coconut milk, and orange juice into a blender.
2. Add ice cubes if you prefer a colder drink.
3. Blend until smooth and transport yourself to a tropical paradise.

# Spinach and Banana Smoothie

Ingredients:

- 2 cups fresh spinach leaves
- 1 banana
- 1/2 cup plain Greek yogurt

- 1/2 cup water
- 1 tablespoon honey
- Ice cubes (optional)

Instructions:

1. Combine spinach, banana, Greek yogurt, water, and honey in a blender.
2. Add ice cubes for a chillier texture.
3. Blend until the mixture is smooth and vibrant.

## Antioxidant Powerhouse Smoothie

Ingredients:

- 1 cup mixed berries (blueberries, blackberries)
- 1/2 cup kale leaves
- 1/2 cup pomegranate juice
- 1/2 cup almond milk
- Ice cubes (optional)

Instructions:

1. Place mixed berries, kale, pomegranate juice, and almond milk in a blender.
2. Add ice cubes for a refreshing twist.

3. Blend until the smoothie is rich in color and flavor.

## Cucumber and Kiwi Cooler

Ingredients:

- 1 cucumber, peeled and chopped
- 2 kiwis, peeled and sliced
- 1/2 lime, juiced
- 1/2 cup water
- 1 tablespoon honey (optional)
- Ice cubes (optional)

Instructions:

1. Add cucumber, kiwis, lime juice, water, and honey to a blender.
2. Include ice cubes for extra freshness.
3. Blend until the mixture is cool and invigorating.

## Peanut Butter Banana Smoothie

Ingredients:

- 2 bananas
- 2 tablespoons peanut butter

- 1 cup almond milk
- 1 tablespoon honey
- Ice cubes (optional)

Instructions:

1. Combine bananas, peanut butter, almond milk, and honey in a blender.
2. Add ice cubes for a frosty texture.
3. Blend until the mixture is smooth and nutty.

## Pineapple and Kale Smoothie

Ingredients:

- 1 cup pineapple chunks
- 1/2 cup kale leaves
- 1/2 cup coconut milk
- 1/2 cup orange juice
- Ice cubes (optional)

Instructions:

1. Place pineapple, kale, coconut milk, and orange juice in a blender.
2. Add ice cubes for a cooler taste.

3.  Blend until the mixture is tropical and green.

## Creamy Almond and Date Smoothie

Ingredients:

- 1/4 cup almonds, soaked and peeled
- 2 dates, pitted
- 1 banana
- 1/2 cup almond milk
- Ice cubes (optional)

Instructions:

1.  Combine soaked almonds, dates, banana, almond milk, and ice cubes in a blender.
2.  Blend until smooth and creamy.

## Blueberry and Oat Smoothie

Ingredients:

- 1 cup blueberries
- 1/4 cup rolled oats
- 1/2 cup Greek yogurt
- 1/2 cup almond milk

- 1 tablespoon honey
- Ice cubes (optional)

Instructions:

1. Add blueberries, rolled oats, Greek yogurt, almond milk, and honey to a blender.
2. Include ice cubes for a refreshing texture.
3. Blend until the mixture is smooth and satisfying.

## Orange Creamsicle Smoothie

Ingredients:

- 1 cup orange segments
- 1/2 cup plain Greek yogurt
- 1/2 cup almond milk
- 1 tablespoon honey
- Ice cubes (optional)

Instructions:

1. Combine orange segments, Greek yogurt, almond milk, and honey in a blender.
2. Add ice cubes for a chillier texture.

3.  Blend until the smoothie is reminiscent of a classic creamsicle.

## Coffee and Oat Smoothie

Ingredients:

- 1/2 cup brewed coffee, cooled
- 1/4 cup rolled oats
- 1/2 banana
- 1/2 cup almond milk
- 1 tablespoon honey
- Ice cubes (optional)

Instructions:

1.  Place cooled coffee, rolled oats, banana, almond milk, and honey into a blender.
2.  Include ice cubes if you prefer it cold.
3.  Blend until the mixture is both energizing and filling.

## Beet and Berry Smoothie

Ingredients:

- 1/2 cup cooked beets, diced

- 1 cup mixed berries (strawberries, raspberries)
- 1/2 cup Greek yogurt
- 1/2 cup water
- 1 tablespoon honey
- Ice cubes (optional)

Instructions:

1. Add cooked beets, mixed berries, Greek yogurt, water, and honey to a blender.
2. For an extra chill, include ice cubes.
3. Blend until the smoothie is both vibrant and nutritious.

## Watermelon and Mint Smoothie

Ingredients:

- 2 cups watermelon, diced
- 5-6 fresh mint leaves
- 1/2 lime, juiced
- 1/2 cup water
- Ice cubes (optional)

Instructions:

1.  Combine watermelon, mint leaves, lime juice, water, and ice cubes in a blender.

2.  Blend until the mixture is refreshingly minty and summery.

## Chia and Mango Smoothie

Ingredients:

- 1 cup mango chunks
- 1/4 cup chia seeds
- 1/2 cup coconut milk
- 1/2 cup almond milk
- 1 tablespoon honey
- Ice cubes (optional)

Instructions:

1.  Place mango chunks, chia seeds, coconut milk, almond milk, and honey into a blender.

2.  For a colder consistency, add ice cubes.

3.  Blend until the smoothie is both rich in flavor and packed with nutrients.

# CONCLUSION

As we close this chapter, we want to remind you that this journey doesn't have an endpoint. It's an ongoing adventure where you're the chef, the artist, and the connoisseur. Maintaining a diet that caters to your specific health needs is a lifelong endeavor. We encourage you to keep exploring, keep experimenting, and keep nurturing your health with every meal you prepare.

We'd like to express our deepest gratitude for joining us on this voyage. We hope that the recipes and insights shared in this cookbook become cherished tools in your journey toward health and happiness. Remember, your health is your most valuable possession, and every choice you make is a step toward preserving it.

In the spirit of health, community, and shared experiences, we close this book, but the kitchen is where your culinary odyssey truly begins. Keep cooking, keep nourishing, and above all, keep savoring the journey of life. Thank you for being a part of our cookbook adventure.